The Easy Anti-inflammatory Diet

Recipes For Stronger Immune System

Lysandra Carter

Disclaimer

The information contained in this book, "The Easy anti-inflammatory diet" is for educational purposes only and is not intended to be a substitute for professional medical advice, diagnosis or treatment. The author is not a medical professional and cannot provide medical advice. Always seek the advice of your physician or other qualified healthcare provider with any questions you may have regarding a medical condition. Never disregard professional medical advice or delay in seeking it because of something you have read in this book.

About the Author

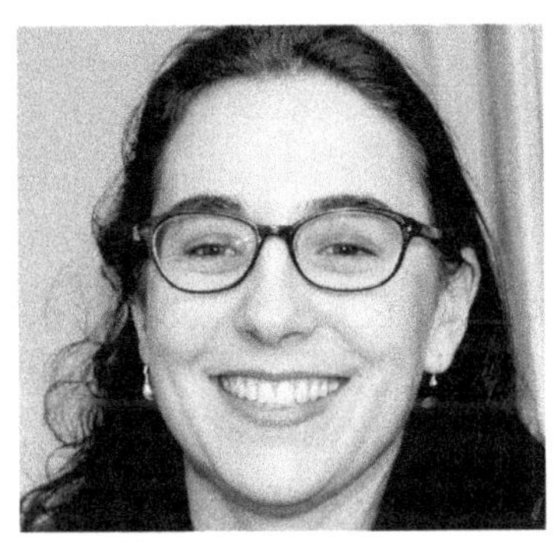 **Lysandra Carter** is not your typical chef; rather, she is a culinary artist who is passionate about producing mouthwatering dishes that encourage a healthy lifestyle in addition to tantalizing the taste sensations. Having a natural passion for food from birth, Lysandra has developed her ability to prepare meals into a potent instrument for enhancing wellbeing.

She has devoted years to perfecting her skills as a chef and learning about the various facets of cooking. Her culinary travels have taken her to several kitchens, ranging from elegant places to small neighborhood eateries. She is known for her ability to creatively combine flavors, textures, and nutritional value in her cooking, which is a result of her dedication to culinary perfection.

What distinguishes Lysandra out is her lifelong interest in healthy eating and lifestyle decisions. In addition to cooking delicious food, she promotes wholesome, well-balanced meals. She thinks that eating is a way to nourish the body, mind, and soul in addition to providing nourishment. Her meals are a delightful blend of nutrition and flavor that elevate healthy eating to a luxurious level.

Apart from her passion for cooking, Lysandra has an active and exciting personal life. Even though she's still unmarried, her love for creating unique experiences goes beyond the kitchen. Lysandra is full of life, and it shows in everything she does, be it cooking alone or spending time with friends and family.

Table Of Contents

Chapter 4: Dinner Favorites

- One-Pot Garlicky Shrimp & Spinach
- One-Pot Chicken & Broccoli Pasta
- Creamy Salmon Pasta with Sun-Dried Tomatoes
- White Bean & Sun-Dried Tomato Gnocchi
- Quinoa Chili with Sweet Potatoes

Chapter 5: Healthy Snacks

- Almond-Stuffed Dates
- Instant-Pot Cashew Yogurt
- Crunchy Roasted Chickpeas
- Sriracha-Buffalo Cauliflower Bites
- Air-Fryer Crispy Chickpeas

Chapter 6: Healthy Drinks

- Green Juice
- Anti-Inflammatory Golden Tonic
- Ginger-Turmeric-Carrot Shots
- Apple Cider Vinegar Tonic
- Elderberry Elixir Mocktail

Chapter 7: Vegetarian Recipes

- Vegan Lentil Soup
- Frittata with Asparagus, Leek & Ricotta
- Guacamole Chopped Salad
- Chhole (Chickpea Curry)
- Quinoa-Black Bean Salad

Review

Introduction

Inflammation protects our bodies against dangers like germs, injuries, and poisons. When our body senses a threat, whether an invading germ or damaged tissue, it triggers inflammation. This process aims to remove the threat and start healing. Acute inflammation is normal and vital. It allows our body to fight infections and repair damaged cells and tissues.

Long-lasting inflammation can cause trouble. It might persist even after the initial threat is gone or when the immune system wrongly attacks healthy tissues. Unlike short-term, localized inflammation, chronic inflammation affects the entire body. It contributes to various chronic diseases developing.

Health issues like heart disease, obesity, diabetes, arthritis, and Crohn's can stem from long-term inflammation. The body's immune system stays active too long. This causes harm and degeneration. Brain diseases like Alzheimer's and some cancers also link to inflammation. Inflammation impacts aging in organs. It leads to deterioration as years pass by. Short sentences vary with long ones to create more burstiness in the content while simple words minimize perplexity levels.

The way chronic inflammation happens involves many complicated things. Your body's immune system, genetics, habits, environment, and health issues interact. Poor eating, inactivity, stress, little sleep, and toxins promote it. Being obese, smoking, and lasting infections make inflammation worse. These raise the chances of getting chronic diseases.

Chronic inflammation affects health a lot. That's why people want to find ways to control inflammation and lower disease risk. One method is changing your diet. You can eat anti-inflammatory foods and avoid inflammatory ones. This helps regulate your body's inflammatory response. It promotes good overall health and wellbeing.

Inflammation has two sides. It protects our bodies, but too much causes harm. It's vital to grasp how inflammation affects health. The right approach includes diet changes, active living, and medical care when needed. Taking these steps supports immune function and reduces risks from chronic inflammation-related diseases.

➢ Benefits of Supporting Immune Health Through Diet

There are several advantages to immune system support through nutrition that go beyond preventing infections and colds. Here's a closer look at the benefits of making immunological health a top priority in your diet:

(a) Enhanced Disease Resistance: A healthy immune system is better able to recognize and get rid of pathogens, which include bacteria, viruses, and other dangerous microbes. A diet high in immune-stimulating foods can help people fortify their defenses and lower their risk of illness.

(b) Faster Recovery: Having a robust immune system helps hasten the healing process in the event of disease or infection. The body recovers from disease or damage more quickly when certain nutrients, like vitamin C, zinc, and protein, are present. These nutrients also play important roles in immune system function and tissue healing.

(c) Reduced Inflammation: Chronic inflammation can weaken the immune system and play a role in the emergence of a number of illnesses, including allergies, metabolic problems, and autoimmune diseases. Numerous dietary components, including antioxidants, phytochemicals, and omega-3 fatty acids, have anti-inflammatory qualities and can aid in reducing inflammation in the body.

(d) Protection Against Chronic Diseases: Numerous chronic conditions, such as heart disease, type 2 diabetes, and some malignancies, have chronic inflammation as one of their common underlying causes. People can lower their chance of getting these illnesses and improve long-term health by eating an anti-inflammatory diet high in fruits, vegetables, whole grains, and healthy fats.

(e) Optimized Gut Health: Immune response is largely dependent on the gut microbiota, where a well-balanced and diversified microbial community plays a key role. A healthy gut microbiota is supported by dietary elements like fiber, prebiotics, and fermented foods, which strengthen the immune system and lower the risk of inflammation and gastrointestinal illnesses.

(f) Improved Mental Well-being: Emerging research suggests that there is a bidirectional relationship between the gut and the brain known as the gut-brain axis. An imbalance in gut microbiota, known as dysbiosis, has been linked to mood disorders such as depression and anxiety. By supporting gut health through diet, individuals may experience improvements in mood and mental well-being.

(g) Improved Mental Well-being: The gut-brain axis is a term used to describe a potentially bidirectional interaction between the gut and the brain, according to emerging studies. Anxiety and depression have been associated with dysbiosis, an imbalance in the gut flora. Those who maintain their gut health with food may see changes in their mental and emotional wellness.

(h) Reduced Healthcare Costs: Long-term healthcare expenditures may be decreased for those who invest in preventive measures like nutritional therapies to enhance immunological health. Reduced rates of chronic illness, fewer infections, and better general health can result in cheaper medical costs and a better standard of living.

In summary, there are several advantages to bolstering immune function through nutrition, including less inflammation and increased resistance to illness, as well as better gut health, longevity, and mental clarity. People can improve their general health and well-being, fortify their body's defenses, lower their chance of developing chronic illnesses, and increase their intake of immune-boosting foods and minerals.

➢ **Overview of the Anti-Inflammatory Diet Approach**

The Anti-Inflammatory Diet Approach is a way of eating that places a focus on eating more foods that have anti-inflammatory qualities and reducing or eliminating items that make inflammation worse. This method is based on the knowledge that a number of diseases, including diabetes, heart disease, arthritis, and some types of cancer, are significantly influenced by chronic inflammation. People can help control inflammation in the body and advance general health and wellbeing by making wise food choices.

An extended overview of the Anti-Inflammatory diet approach is provided below:

Focus on Whole, Nutrient-Dense Foods: Nutrient- and antioxidant-rich whole, minimally processed foods form the cornerstone of the anti-inflammatory diet. Fruits, vegetables, whole grains, legumes, nuts, seeds, and lean proteins are a few of these. A wealth of vitamins, minerals, fiber, and phytochemicals found in whole meals boost the immune system and lower inflammation.

Emphasis on Omega-3 Fatty Acids: Omega-3 fatty acids are found in fatty fish (salmon, mackerel, and sardines), flaxseeds, chia seeds, walnuts, and hemp seeds. They are also recognized to have anti-inflammatory qualities. By balancing the ratio of omega-3 to omega-6 fatty acids in the diet, including sources of omega-3 fatty acids can help reduce inflammation.

Healthy Fats over Saturated and Trans Fats: While reducing the intake of trans and saturated fats, the anti-inflammatory diet promotes the consumption of good fats such those found in nuts, seeds, avocados, and olive oil. Commonly found in processed foods, fried foods, and baked goods, saturated and trans fats have been related to an elevated risk of chronic disease and inflammation.

Colorful Fruits and Vegetables: Antioxidants, vitamins, and minerals found in abundance in fruits and vegetables aid in the body's fight against oxidative stress and inflammation. Fruits and vegetables that have bright hues indicate that they contain phytochemicals with strong anti-inflammatory qualities, like flavonoids and carotenoids.

Herbs and Spices: It has been demonstrated that several herbs and spices have potent anti-inflammatory qualities. Spices that can be added to food to improve flavor and reduce inflammation include turmeric, ginger, garlic, cinnamon, and cloves.

Minimize Processed Foods and Added Sugars: Foods that have been processed, especially those that are heavy in harmful fats, artificial additives, and refined sugars, can cause inflammation in the body. The Anti-Inflammatory Diet suggests consuming more whole, nutrient-dense meals and minimizing or avoiding processed foods and sugary drinks.

Hydration: Maintaining hydration is crucial for promoting general health and lowering inflammatory levels. The greatest option for being hydrated is water, however herbal teas and infused water can also help you stay hydrated and provide extra antioxidant benefits.

Individualized Approach: It's critical to understand that there is no one-size-fits-all Anti-Inflammatory Diet. Different people may react differently to different foods, and depending on personal preferences, food sensitivities, and medical conditions, dietary adjustments may be required.

In conclusion, studies have demonstrated that eating full, nutrient-rich foods can lower inflammation and strengthen the immune system. This is why the Anti-Inflammatory Diet Approach is advocated. People can take preventative measures to control inflammation, lower their chance of developing chronic illnesses, and improve their general health by following this dietary pattern.

Chapter One

The Anti-Inflammatory Diet is a way of eating that emphasizes avoiding foods that aggravate inflammation in the body and ingesting those that are known to lessen it. The focus is on complete, high-nutrient foods such fruits, vegetables, whole grains, nuts, seeds, and healthy fats like those in olive oil and fatty fish. Reducing processed foods, refined carbohydrates, and harmful fats is another recommendation of the diet. People who adhere to this dietary pattern want to control inflammation, lower their chance of developing chronic illnesses, and improve their general health and wellbeing.

The body's immune system naturally and critically responds to damaging stimuli, such as infections, wounds, or irritants, by producing inflammation. The body launches an inflammatory reaction to counteract a threat and aid in healing when it senses one, whether it be a bacterial or viral infection, a physical wound, or exposure to toxins. At the location of the injury or infection, this acute inflammation is characterized by redness, swelling, heat, and discomfort. Usually, this inflammation goes away once the threat has been removed or the healing process has started.

But if inflammation lasts for a long period or develops into a chronic condition, it may become troublesome. Chronic inflammation arises when the immune system gets dysregulated and unintentionally targets healthy tissues, or when the inflammatory response persists even after the original threat has been eliminated. In contrast to acute inflammation, which is a transient and limited reaction, chronic inflammation can impact the entire body and play a role in the emergence of a number of medical disorders.

1.1 Here are some ways that inflammation impacts the body's many systems:

Cardiovascular System: The onset and advancement of cardiovascular disorders, including atherosclerosis (hardening of the arteries), coronary artery disease, and stroke, have been linked to chronic inflammation. Inflammation can cause harm to the blood vessel's inner lining, encourage the accumulation of plaque, and cause the arteries to constrict, which lowers blood flow and raises the risk of a heart attack or stroke.

Metabolic System: Chronic inflammation is strongly associated with metabolic disorders, including obesity, insulin resistance, and type 2 diabetes. Inflammation can impair glucose metabolism and insulin resistance by interfering with the body's ability to regulate blood sugar levels. It can also cause hormonal imbalance and the release of pro-inflammatory cytokines from adipose (fat) tissue, which exacerbates metabolic dysfunction.

Musculoskeletal System: Chronic inflammation in the joints can result in pain, stiffness, and decreased mobility. Rheumatoid arthritis, osteoarthritis, and autoimmune disorders like lupus are examples of inflammatory conditions that cause this. Over time, inflammation can lead to joint deterioration and a decline in function by causing damage to bone and cartilage.

Digestive System: Crohn's disease, ulcerative colitis, and other inflammatory bowel diseases (IBD) can be brought on by persistent inflammation of the gastrointestinal system. Inflammation can cause harm to the intestinal lining, which can result in nutritional malabsorption, diarrhea, bleeding in the rectal area, and stomach pain.

Immune System: Dysregulated inflammation can weaken the immune system and make people more vulnerable to allergies, autoimmune illnesses, and infections. The equilibrium of immune cells and cytokines can be upset by chronic inflammation, which can result in an overactive or underactive immune response.

Central Nervous System: Neurodegenerative illnesses like multiple sclerosis, Parkinson's disease, and Alzheimer's disease have been linked to inflammation in the central nervous system. Inflammatory processes have the potential to harm neurons, interfere with brain signaling, and accelerate the development of neurological conditions.

The main idea behind anti-inflammatory eating is to limit or stay away from meals that have been demonstrated to increase inflammation in the body while consuming

nutrients that have been proven to decrease inflammation.

1.2 An explanation of these ideas is provided below:

Emphasize Whole, Nutrient-Dense Foods: The Anti-Inflammatory diet is based mostly on whole foods, including fruits, vegetables, whole grains, legumes, nuts, seeds, and lean proteins. These foods are abundant in antioxidants, phytochemicals, vitamins, and minerals that boost immunity and reduce inflammation.

Include healthy fats: An important aspect of the Anti-Inflammatory diet are healthy fats, especially those found in fatty fish (including salmon, mackerel, and sardines), avocado, nuts, and seeds, as well as olive oil. In particular, omega-3 fatty acids have strong anti-inflammatory qualities and can aid in lowering inflammation in the body.

Prioritize Omega-3 Fatty Acids: Since the body cannot create omega-3 fatty acids on its own, it is necessary to consume them through diet. Walnuts, hemp seeds, chia seeds, flaxseeds, and fatty fish (salmon, trout, and sardines) are good sources of omega-3 fatty acids. By balancing the diet's omega-3 to omega-6 fatty acid ratio, consuming these foods can help lower inflammation.

Load Up on colorful fruits and vegetables: Antioxidants, vitamins, and minerals found in abundance in fruits and vegetables aid in the body's fight against oxidative stress and inflammation. Fruits and vegetables that have bright hues indicate that they contain phytochemicals with strong anti-inflammatory qualities, like flavonoids and carotenoids.

Incorporate Herbs and Spices: It has been demonstrated that several herbs and spices have potent anti-inflammatory qualities. Spices that can be added to food to improve flavor and reduce inflammation include turmeric, ginger, garlic, cinnamon, and cloves.

Limit Processed Foods and Added Sugars: Foods that have been processed, especially those that are heavy in harmful fats, artificial additives, and refined sugars, can cause inflammation in the body. The Anti-Inflammatory Diet suggests consuming more whole, nutrient-dense meals and minimizing or avoiding processed foods and sugary drinks.

Stay Hydrated: Maintaining hydration is crucial for promoting general health and lowering inflammatory levels. The best option for being hydrated is water, however herbal teas and infused water can also help you stay hydrated and provide extra antioxidant benefits.

Individualize Your Approach: It's critical to understand that there is no one-size-fits-all Anti-Inflammatory Diet. Different people may react differently to different foods, and depending on personal preferences, food sensitivities, and medical conditions, dietary adjustments may be required. You can customize the diet to fit your specific needs by trying different things and paying attention to your body's signals.

Individuals can make educated dietary decisions to help control inflammation, lower their chance of developing chronic illnesses, and improve their general health and well-being by adhering to these anti-inflammatory eating practices.

It is impossible to exaggerate the significance of immune support in the diet as the foods we eat have a profound impact on how our immune systems function and how well our bodies function as a whole.

1.3 Here's more information on the importance of immunological support in the diet:

Enhanced Disease Resistance: An immune system that receives proper support is more capable of recognizing and getting rid of pathogens, including bacteria, viruses, and other dangerous microbes. A number of nutrients, including antioxidants, zinc, vitamin C, and vitamin D, are essential for immunological function and help fortify the body's resistance to diseases and infections.

Faster Recovery from Illness: A strong immune system speeds up healing in the event of disease or infection. Vitamin C, zinc, and protein are among the nutrients that help the body heal from disease, injury, or surgery more quickly by supporting tissue repair and immunological function.

Reduced Risk of Chronic Diseases: In addition, a robust immune system is essential for warding against chronic illnesses like diabetes, cancer, heart disease, and autoimmune diseases. These illnesses are associated with oxidative stress and chronic inflammation, both of which can be brought on by immune system malfunction. People can lower their chance of developing chronic illnesses and increase their longevity and vitality by eating a diet that supports immunological health.

Balanced Inflammation Response: An important part of controlling inflammation in the body is the immune system. While inflammation is a normal and essential reaction to an infection or injury, prolonged inflammation can also play a role in the emergence of a number of diseases. A balanced and robust immune system can be supported by modifying the body's inflammatory response to certain nutrients and bioactive chemicals included in food.

Optimized Gut Health: The trillions of bacteria that reside in the gastrointestinal system and make up the gut microbiota are essential for immunological function. Immune health is supported by a diversified and well-balanced gut microbiota that reduces inflammation, boosts antibody production, and guards against infections. Eating a diet high in fiber, probiotics, and prebiotics helps to maintain a healthy gut flora, which boosts immunity and lowers the risk of inflammation and gastrointestinal illnesses.

Stress Management: Chronic stress can weaken the immune system and increase susceptibility to infections and illnesses. Certain nutrients, such as vitamin C, vitamin B6, and magnesium, support adrenal function and help the body cope with stress. Additionally, foods rich in omega-3 fatty acids, antioxidants, and phytochemicals have been shown to reduce stress-related inflammation and support overall resilience to stress.

Overall Health and Well-being: People can enhance their general health and well-being by enhancing their immune system through nutrition. The critical vitamins, minerals, antioxidants, and phytochemicals required to enhance immune function, lower inflammation, and promote optimal health and vitality can be found in a wide variety of nutrient-dense foods that are balanced and diverse in their diet.

In conclusion, it is critical to include immune-boosting foods in the diet in order to improve disease resistance, encourage quicker healing from illnesses, lower the chance of developing chronic illnesses, balance inflammation, improve gut health, handle stress, and promote general health and wellbeing. People can improve resilience to sickness, fortify their body's defenses, and live longer by giving priority to foods and nutrients that build the immune system in their diet.

Chapter Two: Breakfast Recipes

2.1 Spinach & Egg Scramble with Raspberries

This quick egg scramble with hearty bread is one of the best anti-inflammatory breakfast foods. It combines protein-packed eggs and superfood raspberries with filling whole-grain toast and nutrient-rich spinach. The protein and fiber help fill you up and keep you going through the morning.

Preparation Information

Prep Time:10 mins

Total Time:10 mins

Servings:1

Yield:1 serving

Nutritional Information

Servings Per Recipe: 1

Serving Size: 2 eggs, 1 slice bread & 1/2 cup raspberries

Calories: 296

Total Carbohydrate: 21g

Dietary Fiber: 7g

Total Sugars: 5g

Protein: 18g

Total Fat: 16g

Saturated Fat: 4g

Cholesterol: 372mg

Vitamin A: 3313IU

Vitamin C: 28mg

Folate: 79 mcg

Sodium: 394mg

Calcium: 139mg

Iron: 4mg

Magnesium: 76mg

Potassium: 293mg

Ingredients

1 teaspoon canola oil

1 ½ cups baby spinach (1 1/2 ounces)

2 large eggs, lightly beaten

Pinch of kosher salt

Pinch of ground pepper

1 slice whole-grain bread, toasted

½ cup fresh raspberries

Directions

- Heat oil in a small nonstick skillet over medium-high heat. Add spinach and cook until wilted, stirring often, 1 to 2 minutes. Transfer the spinach to a plate. Wipe the pan clean, place over medium heat and add eggs. Cook, stirring once or twice to ensure even cooking, until just set, 1 to 2 minutes. Stir in the spinach, salt and pepper. Serve the scramble with toast and raspberries.

2.2 Smoked Salmon & Cream Cheese Omelet

The key to this healthy smoked salmon omelet recipe is cooking the eggs over low heat so the curds set up nice and soft. A splash of milk in the eggs is added insurance to keep the salmon omelet from turning rubbery.

Preparation Information

Cook Time:15 mins

Total Time:15 mins

Servings:1

Yield:1 serving

Nutritional Information

Servings Per Recipe: 1

Calories: 254

Total Carbohydrate: 3g

Dietary Fiber: 0g

Total Sugars: 2g

Protein: 17g

Total Fat: 19g

Saturated Fat: 9g

Cholesterol: 402mg

Vitamin A: 901IU

Vitamin C: 1mg

Folate: 52mcg

Sodium: 458mg

Calcium: 84mg

Iron: 2mg

Magnesium: 19mg

Potassium: 217mg

Ingredients

2 large eggs

1 teaspoon reduced-fat milk or water

⅛ teaspoon ground pepper, plus more for garnish

Pinch of salt

1 teaspoon butter

2 tablespoons chopped smoked salmon

1 tablespoon cream cheese, softened, or crumbled feta

1 tablespoon finely chopped red onion

1 ½ teaspoons chopped fresh dill, plus more for garnish

Directions

- Whisk eggs, milk (or water), pepper and salt in a small bowl.

- Melt butter in a small nonstick skillet over medium-low heat, tilting the pan to make sure the entire bottom is coated. Add the egg mixture and cook for 1 minute without stirring. Sprinkle salmon, cheese, onion and dill over one half of the eggs. Cook for 1 minute. Using a flexible spatula, lift the bare side to let raw egg from the middle flow underneath; you may need to tilt the pan slightly. Continue lifting in different spots until there's almost no raw egg on top. Cook for 2 minutes or more.

- Using the spatula, flip the bare side over the filling, folding the omelet in half, and cook for 1 minute. (If the eggs are starting to brown, lower the heat.) Carefully flip the omelet over and cook 1 minute more. Serve immediately, garnished with more dill and pepper, if desired.

2.3 Avocado & Kale Omelet

This omelet with avocado and kale is a filling, high-protein breakfast. With its high fiber content, kale helps stave off hunger for longer in this nutritious omelet recipe.

Preparation Information

Prep Time:10 mins

Total Time:10 mins

Servings:1

Yield:1 serving

Nutritional Information

Servings Per Recipe: 1

Serving Size: 1 omelet

Calories: 339

Total Carbohydrate: 9g

Dietary Fiber: 4g

Total Sugars: 2g

Protein: 15g

Total Fa:t 28g

Saturated Fat: 6g

Cholesterol: 372mg

Vitamin A: 2343IU

Vitamin C: 29mg

Folate: 119mcg

Sodium: 446mg

Calcium: 97mg

Iron: 3mg

Magnesium: 40mg

Potassium: 506mg

Ingredients

2 large eggs

1 teaspoon low-fat milk

Pinch of salt

2 teaspoons extra-virgin olive oil, divided

1 cup chopped kale

1 tablespoon lime juice

1 tablespoon chopped fresh cilantro

1 teaspoon unsalted sunflower seeds

Pinch of crushed red pepper

Pinch of salt

¼ avocado, sliced

Directions

- Beat eggs with milk and salt in a small bowl. Heat 1 teaspoon oil in a small nonstick skillet over medium heat. Add the egg mixture and cook until the bottom is set and the center is still a bit runny, 1 to 2 minutes. Flip the omelet over and cook until set, about 30 seconds more. Transfer to a plate.

- Toss kale with the remaining 1 teaspoon oil, lime juice, cilantro, sunflower seeds, crushed red pepper and a pinch of salt. Top the omelet with the kale salad and avocado.

2.4 Mango & Kale Smoothie

The blend of kale, mango, banana and orange juice gives this healthy smoothie an extra-fresh and tropical flavor profile.

Preparation Information

Active Time:10 mins

Total Time:10 mins

Servings:1

Nutritional Information

Servings Per Recipe: 1

Serving Size: about 2 cups

Calories: 329

Total Carbohydrate: 82g

Dietary Fiber: 6g

Total Sugars: 62g

Protein: 4g

Total Fat: 1g

Vitamin A: 3492IU

Sodium: 10mg

Potassium: 936mg

Ingredients

1 cup baby kale

1 cup frozen mango chunks

1 small banana, sliced

1 cup fresh orange juice

Directions

- Add kale, mango, banana and orange juice to a blender. Blend on medium-low speed, using the tamper as necessary, until well combined.

- Increase speed to medium-high and blend until very smooth.

2.5 Smoked Trout & Spinach Scrambled Eggs

Elevate plain-Jane scrambled eggs with smoked trout and fresh spinach in this healthy breakfast recipe.

Preparation Information

Prep Time:15 mins

Total Time:15 mins

Servings:2

Nutritional Information

Servings Per Recipe: 2

Serving Size: about 3/4 cup each

Calories: 243

Total Carbohydrate: 4g

Dietary Fiber: 1g

Total Sugars: 2g

Protein: 19g

Total Fat: 17g

Saturated Fat: 4g

Cholesterol: 379mg

Vitamin A: 2096IU

Vitamin C: 5mg

Folate: 80mcg

Sodium: 455mg

Calcium: 94mg

Iron: 2mg

Magnesium: 28mg

Potassium: 280mg

Ingredients

4 large eggs

2 tablespoons reduced-fat milk

¼ teaspoon ground pepper

Pinch of salt

2 teaspoons grapeseed oil or avocado oil

2 tablespoons finely chopped shallot

½ cup boned and flaked smoked trout (1 1/2 ounces)

1 cup chopped spinach

Instructions

- Whisk eggs, milk, pepper and salt in a medium bowl until pale yellow throughout.

- Heat oil in a medium nonstick skillet over medium heat. Add shallot and cook, stirring, until starting to brown, 1 to 2 minutes. Add the egg mixture and reduce heat to medium-low. Cook, undisturbed, until the edges start to set, about 30 seconds. Sprinkle trout over the eggs. Using a rubber spatula, gently push and fold the eggs until fluffy and barely set, 2 to 4 minutes. Stir in spinach. Remove from heat, cover and let stand until the spinach is just wilted, 1 to 2 minutes.

Chapter 3: Lunch ideas

3.1 Smoked Trout & Spinach Scrambled Eggs

Preparation Information

Prep Time:15 mins

Total Time: 15 mins

Servings: 2

Yield: 2 serving

Nutritional Information

Servings Per Recipe: 2

Serving Size: about 3/4 cup each

Calories: 243

Total Carbohydrate: 4g

Dietary Fiber: 1g

Total Sugars: 2g

Protein: 19g

Total Fat: 17g

Saturated Fat: 4g

Cholesterol: 379mg

Vitamin A: 2096IU

Vitamin C: 5mg

Folate: 80mcg

Sodium: 455mg

Calcium: 94mg

Iron: 2mg

Magnesium: 28mg

Potassium: 280mg

Ingredients

4 large eggs

2 tablespoons reduced-fat milk

¼ teaspoon ground pepper

Pinch of salt

2 teaspoons grapeseed oil or avocado oil

2 tablespoons finely chopped shallot

½ cup boned and flaked smoked trout (1 1/2 ounces)

1 cup chopped spinach

Instructions

- Whisk eggs, milk, pepper and salt in a medium bowl until pale yellow throughout.

- Heat oil in a medium nonstick skillet over medium heat. Add shallot and cook, stirring, until starting to brown, 1 to 2 minutes. Add the egg mixture and reduce heat to medium-low. Cook, undisturbed, until the edges start to set, about 30 seconds. Sprinkle trout over the eggs. Using a rubber spatula, gently push and fold the eggs until fluffy and barely set, 2 to 4 minutes. Stir in spinach. Remove from heat, cover and let stand until the spinach is just wilted, 1 to 2 minutes.

3.2 Cucumber-Chicken Green Goddess Wrap

This quick and easy wrap rolls up and is ready for a casual, stationary lunch or a meal on the go, with protein from chicken to keep you going. The green goddess dressing is creamy with cheese and avocado and bright from lemon and herbs. Cucumber and carrots add color and crunch to this healthy, robust whole-wheat wrap.

Preparation Information

Active Time:

10 mins

Total Time:

10 mins

Servings:

1

Nutritional Information (per serving)

Servings Per Recipe: 1

Serving Size: 1 wrap

Calories: 353

Total Carbohydrate: 28g

Dietary Fiber: 6g

Total Sugars: 3g

Protein: 18g

Total Fat: 19g

Saturated Fat: 7g

Cholesterol: 58mg

Vitamin A: 4102IU

Vitamin C: 23mg

Vitamin D: 2IU

Vitamin E: 2mg

Folate: 93mcg

Vitamin K: 141mcg

Sodium: 590mg

Calcium: 123mg

Iron: 2mg

Magnesium: 44mg

Potassium: 591mg

Zinc: 1mg

Ingredients

1 ounce cream cheese, at room temperature

¼ medium avocado, mashed

1 teaspoon lemon juice or rice vinegar

⅛ teaspoon salt

⅛ teaspoon ground pepper

2 tablespoons chopped fresh herbs such as parsley, dill and/or basil

1 (8 inch) whole-wheat tortilla

¼ cup shredded cooked chicken

2 tablespoons shredded carrot

6 thin slices cucumber

½ cup mixed salad greens

Instructions

- Stir cream cheese, avocado, lemon juice (or vinegar), salt and pepper together in a small bowl. Add herbs and stir until well blended. Spread the mixture evenly on tortilla. Top with chicken, carrot, cucumber and greens, then roll up like a burrito.

3.3 Lemony Lentil Salad with Feta

This delicious and healthy lentil salad comes together in just 30 minutes and makes a wonderful hot-weather meal. Serve with whole-wheat pitas, if desired.

Preparation Information

Cook Time: 30 mins

Total Time: 30 mins

Servings: 6

Yield: 6 servings, 1 cup each

Nutritional Information

Servings Per Recipe: 6

Calories: 280

Total Carbohydrate: 24g

Dietary Fiber: 11g

Total Sugars: 4g

Protein: 13g

Total Fat: 16g

Saturated Fat: 4g

Cholesterol: 7mg

Vitamin A: 812IU

Vitamin C: 35mg

Folate: 16mcg

Sodium: 536mg

Calcium: 98mg

Iron: 3mg

Magnesium: 7mg

Potassium: 108mg

Ingredients

⅓ cup lemon juice

⅓ cup chopped fresh dill

2 teaspoons Dijon mustard

¼ teaspoon salt, or to taste

⅓ cup extra-virgin olive oil

Freshly ground pepper, to taste

2 15-ounce cans lentils, rinsed, or 3 cups cooked brown or green lentils

1 cup crumbled feta cheese, (about 4 ounces)

1 medium red bell pepper, seeded and diced (about 1 cup)

1 cup diced seedless cucumber

½ cup finely chopped red onion

Instructions

- Whisk lemon juice, dill, mustard, salt and pepper in a large bowl. Gradually Whisk in oil. Add lentils, feta, bell pepper, cucumber and onion; toss to coat.

3.4 Chickpea Tuna Salad

This salad is a wonderful alternative to traditional tuna salad, offering a boost of plant-based protein and fiber.

Preparation Information

Net Carbs: Net carbs per serving (assuming 4 servings): Approximately 20-21g net carbs per serving

Preparation Time:

Approximately 15-20 minutes

Cook Time:

No cooking required

Nutritional Information

Calories: 200-250 calories

Protein: 15-20 grams

Fat: 7-10 grams

Carbohydrates: 20-25 grams

Dietary Fiber: 5-7 grams

Sugars: 3-5 grams

Sodium: 350-400 milligrams

Ingredients

1 can (15 oz) chickpeas (garbanzo beans), drained and rinsed

1 can (5 oz) tuna in water, drained

1/4 cup diced red onion

1/4 cup diced celery

1/4 cup diced bell pepper (any color)

1/4 cup chopped fresh parsley

2 tablespoons mayonnaise (or Greek yogurt for a lighter option)

1 tablespoon Dijon mustard

1 tablespoon lemon juice

Salt and pepper to taste

Instructions

- Prepare Ingredients:

Drain and rinse the chickpeas well. Use a colander and cold tap water. Drain the canned tuna as well

Dice the red onion, celery, and bell pepper into small, even pieces. Finely chop the fresh parsley.

- Combine Ingredients:

In a large mixing bowl, add the drained and rinsed chickpeas, drained tuna, diced red onion, celery, bell pepper, and chopped parsley.

- Make Dressing:

In a small bowl, whisk together the mayonnaise (or Greek yogurt), Dijon mustard, and lemon juice until smooth and well combined.

- Mix Salad:

Pour the prepared dressing over the ingredients in the mixing bowl.

- Season:

Season the salad with salt and pepper to taste.

- Mix Thoroughly:

Gently toss all the ingredients together until evenly coated with the dressing. Be careful not to mash the chickpeas too much, as they add texture to the salad.

- Chill (Optional):

Cover the bowl with plastic wrap or transfer the salad to an airtight container. Refrigerate for at least 30 minutes to allow the flavors to meld together.

- Serve:

Serve the Chickpea Tuna Salad chilled as desired. It can be enjoyed on its own as a light meal, as a sandwich filling, wrapped in lettuce leaves, or served atop a bed of mixed greens.

3.5 Fall Chopped Salad with Spinach, Butternut Squash, Apples & Cheddar

Who says spinach salads are only for spring? Use autumn's tender crop of fresh spinach and other seasonal vegetables to make this fall salad with roasted butternut squash, apples, cheddar and pecans. This colorful and healthy salad would be a wonderful addition to your Thanksgiving menu, but there's no reason to save it for holidays--serve it along with chicken or pork for a healthy weeknight dinner, or turn it into a main course by adding some chickpeas or chopped chicken or turkey.

Preparation Information

Prep Time: 30 mins

Additional Time: 10 mins

Total Time: 40 mins

Servings: 8

Yield: 10 cups

Nutritional Information

Servings Per Recipe: 8

Serving Size: 1 1/4 cups

Calories: 185

Total Carbohydrate: 16g

Dietary Fiber: 4g

Total Sugars: 5g

Added Sugars: 1g

Protein: 5g

Total Fat: 13g

Saturated Fat: 3g

Cholesterol: 7mg

Vitamin A: 11195IU

Vitamin C: 32mg

Folate: 23mcg

Sodium: 255mg

Calcium: 148mg

Iron: 3mg

Magnesium: 76mg

Potassium: 315mg

Ingredients

1 small (1 1/2 pounds) butternut squash, peeled and cut into 1/2-inch dice (about 4 cups)

2 cloves garlic, minced

3 tablespoons extra-virgin olive oil, divided

½ teaspoon salt, divided

½ teaspoon ground pepper, divided

2 tablespoons balsamic vinegar

1 teaspoon maple syrup

2 teaspoons Dijon mustard

8 cups packed baby spinach, roughly chopped

1 medium Honeycrisp apple, diced

½ cup diced sharp Cheddar cheese

½ cup toasted chopped pecans

Instructions

- Preheat the oven to 400°F. Stir squash, garlic, 1 tablespoon oil, 1/4 teaspoon salt and 1/4 teaspoon pepper together in a large bowl. Spread on a large rimmed baking sheet and roast, stirring once, until tender, about 20 minutes.

- Meanwhile, whisk the remaining 2 tablespoons oil, vinegar, maple syrup, mustard and the remaining 1/4 teaspoon each salt and pepper in the large bowl. Add spinach, the roasted squash, apples, cheese and pecans. Toss to coat.

Chapter 4: Dinner Favorites

4.1 One-Pot Garlicky Shrimp & Spinach

Quick cooking and browning of shrimp, spinach, and garlic make this a great weeknight meal in a pot. Herby parsley, heated crushed red pepper, and zesty lemon juice liven up a quick pan sauce. Serve with a piece of whole-wheat bread so that you can mop up any remaining sauce.

Preparation Information

Active Time: 25 mins

Total Time: 25 mins

Servings: 4

Yield: 4 cups

Nutritional Information

Calories: 226

Fat: 12g

Carbs: 6g

Protein: 26g

Ingredients

3 tablespoons extra-virgin olive oil, divided

6 medium cloves garlic, sliced, divided

1 pound spinach

¼ teaspoon salt plus 1/8 teaspoon, divided

1 tablespoon lemon juice

1 pound shrimp (21-30 count), peeled and deveined

¼ teaspoon crushed red pepper

1 tablespoon finely chopped fresh parsley

1 ½ teaspoons lemon zest

Instructions

- Heat 1 tablespoon of oil in a large pot over medium heat. Add half the garlic and cook until beginning to brown, 1 to 2 minutes. Add spinach and 1/4 teaspoon salt and toss to coat. Cook, stirring once or twice, until mostly wilted, 3 to 5 minutes. Remove from heat and stir in lemon juice. Transfer to a bowl and keep warm.

- Increase heat to medium-high and add the remaining 2 tablespoons oil to the pot. Add the remaining garlic and cook until beginning to brown, 1 to 2 minutes. Add shrimp, crushed red pepper and the remaining 1/8 teaspoon salt; cook, stirring, until the shrimp are just cooked through, 3 to 5 minutes more. Serve the shrimp over the spinach, sprinkled with lemon zest and parsley.

4.2 One-Pot Chicken & Broccoli Pasta

This spaghetti with creamy chicken and broccoli is a simple and quick weeknight meal. In this dish, we use little shells, but you could use orecchiette or any other small pasta.

Preparation Information

Active Time: 20 mins

Total Time: 20 mins

Servings: 4

Nutritional Information

Servings Per Recipe: 4

Serving Size about: 2 cups

Calories: 530

Total Carbohydrate: 52g

Dietary Fiber: 8g

Total Sugars: 7g

Protein: 44g

Total Fat: 18g

Saturated Fat: 6g

Cholesterol: 77mg

Vitamin A: 2769IU

Sodium: 625mg

Potassium: 891mg

Ingredients

2 cups unsalted chicken broth

2 cups water

8 ounces whole-grain small shell pasta

2 tablespoons extra-virgin olive oil

1 ½ tablespoons Worcestershire sauce

1 tablespoon unsalted tomato paste

3 cloves garlic, minced

½ teaspoon ground pepper

¼ teaspoon salt

12 ounces broccoli florets, cut into bite-size pieces

2 cups shredded cooked chicken breast

¾ cup whole-milk plain Greek yogurt

¾ cup grated Parmesan cheese, divided

2 tablespoons chopped fresh dill

Instructions

- Combine broth, water, pasta, oil, Worcestershire, tomato paste, garlic, pepper and salt in a large pot or high-sided skillet. Bring to a boil over high heat, stirring occasionally. Add broccoli; cook, stirring often to prevent the pasta from sticking, until the pasta is al dente, the broccoli is tender and the sauce is creamy, 7 to 8 minutes.

- Remove from heat, and stir in chicken, yogurt, Parmesan and dill.

4.3 Creamy Salmon Pasta with Sun-Dried Tomatoes

There are two ways to use sun-dried tomatoes in this recipe for creamy salmon pasta. Shallots are sautéed in the aromatic oil and then added to the cream sauce with the tomatoes.

Preparation Information

Active Time: 20 mins

Total Time: 25 mins

Servings: 6

Nutritional Information

Servings Per Recipe: 6

Serving Size: about 1 1/2 cups

Calories: 458

Total Carbohydrate: 60g

Dietary Fiber: 8g

Total Sugars: 4g

Protein: 27g

Total Fat: 14g

Saturated Fat: 3g

Cholesterol: 47mg

Vitamin A: 925IU

Sodium: 462mg

Potassium: 867mg

Ingredients

1 pound whole-wheat rigatoni

¼ cup oil-packed sun-dried tomatoes, chopped, plus 2 tablespoons oil from the jar
(or 2 tablespoons olive oil), divided

1 large shallot, finely chopped

2 cloves garlic, minced

½ cup half-and-half

½ cup unsalted chicken broth or vegetable broth

1 teaspoon salt

1 ½ cups loosely packed fresh basil leaves

12 ounces cooked salmon or canned salmon, flaked into 1-inch pieces

2 tablespoons lemon juice

¼ cup chopped fresh flat-leaf parsley

Instructions

- Put a pot of water on to boil. Cook pasta according to package directions to 1 minute before al dente; drain and set aside.

- Meanwhile, heat sun-dried tomato oil (or olive oil) in a large nonstick skillet over medium-high heat. Add shallot and garlic; cook, stirring often, until the shallot is translucent, about 1 minute. Add sun-dried tomatoes, half-and-half, broth and salt. Bring to a simmer over medium-high heat. Reduce heat to medium; cook, stirring occasionally, until thickened and reduced slightly, 5 to 7 minutes.

- Add the pasta to the tomato mixture in the pan. Cook over medium heat, stirring constantly to evenly coat the pasta, for 2 minutes. Stir in basil. Remove from heat. Gently fold in salmon and lemon juice. Sprinkle with parsley and serve.

4.4 White Bean & Sun-Dried Tomato Gnocchi

Sun-dried tomatoes are the star of this recipe—providing texture and umami. Combined with the spinach, they make this dish a great source of vitamins C and K.

Preparation Information

Active Time: 20 mins

Total Time: 20 mins

Servings: 4

Nutritional Information

Servings Per Recipe: 4

Serving Size: 1 cup

Calories: 437

Total Carbohydrate: 69g

Dietary Fiber: 8g

Total Sugars: 4g

Protein: 14g

Total Fat: 13g

Saturated Fat: 5g

Cholesterol: 23mg

Vitamin A: 2995IU

Sodium: 651mg

Potassium: 481mg

Ingredients

½ cup sliced oil-packed sun-dried tomatoes plus 2 tablespoons oil from the jar, divided

1 (16 ounce) package shelf-stable gnocchi

1 (15 ounce) can low-sodium cannellini beans, rinsed

1 (5 ounce) package baby spinach

1 large shallot, minced

⅓ cup low-sodium no-chicken broth or chicken broth

⅓ cup heavy cream

1 tablespoon lemon juice

¼ teaspoon salt

¼ teaspoon ground pepper

3 tablespoons fresh basil leaves

Instructions

- Heat 1 tablespoon of oil in a large nonstick skillet over medium-high heat. Add gnocchi and cook, stirring often, until plumped and starting to brown, about 5 minutes. Add beans and spinach and cook until the spinach is wilted, about 1 minute. Transfer to a plate.

- Add the remaining 1 tablespoon oil to the pan and heat over medium heat. Add sun-dried tomatoes and shallot; cook, stirring, for 1 minute. Increase heat to high and add broth. Cook until the liquid has mostly evaporated, about 2 minutes.

- Reduce heat to medium and stir in cream, lemon juice, salt and pepper. Return the gnocchi mixture to the pan and stir to coat with the sauce. Serve topped with basil.

4.5 Quinoa Chili with Sweet Potatoes

This hearty vegetarian quinoa chili with sweet potatoes has mild spice from poblanos and green chiles. Chili powder, cumin and garlic provide classic chili flavor.

Preparation Information

Active Time: 15 mins

Total Time: 30 mins

Servings: 5

Nutritional Information

Servings Per Recipe: 5

Serving Size: 2 cups

Calories: 346

Total Carbohydrate: 63g

Dietary Fiber: 11g

Total Sugars: 11g

Protein: 12g

Total Fat: 6g

Saturated Fat: 1g

Vitamin A: 10763IU

Sodium: 703mg

Potassium: 862mg

Ingredients

1 tablespoon extra-virgin olive oil

2 (12 ounce) sweet potatoes, peeled and cut into 1/2-inch pieces

1 medium yellow onion, diced

2 poblano peppers, diced

4 large cloves garlic, chopped

1 tablespoon chili powder

2 teaspoons ground cumin

4 cups unsalted vegetable broth

1 (10 ounce) can no-salt-added diced tomatoes with green chiles

1 (4 ounce) can diced green chiles

2 cups water, divided

1 cup uncooked white or multicolored quinoa

1 (15 ounce) can no-salt-added pinto beans, rinsed

½ teaspoon salt

Sliced jalapeño peppers, yogurt and cilantro for serving

Instructions

- Heat oil in a large pot over medium-high heat. Add sweet potatoes and cook, stirring occasionally, until slightly softened and lightly charred, 6 to 7 minutes. Add onion and poblanos; cook, stirring occasionally, until slightly softened, about 3 minutes. Add garlic, chili powder and cumin; cook, stirring constantly, until fragrant, about 30 seconds. Add broth, tomatoes, green chiles and 1 cup water. Cover, increase heat to high and bring to a boil.

- Stir in quinoa, beans and salt. Reduce heat to medium, cover and simmer, stirring occasionally, until the quinoa is tender, about 15 minutes, adding the remaining 1 cup water during the last 3 minutes of cook time. Garnish with jalapeño slices, yogurt and cilantro, if desired.

Chapter 5: Healthy Snacks

5.1 Almond-Stuffed Dates

Medjool dates are softer than their semi-dry Deglet Noor cousins and therefore, much easier to stuff with almonds. This healthy snack recipe can also be turned into an addictive appetizer by adding a little blue cheese to the stuffing.

Preparation Information

Cook Time:5 mins

Total Time:5 mins

Servings:1

Yield:1 serving

Nutritional Information

Servings Per Recipe: 1

Serving Size: 2 stuffed dates

Calories: 149

Total Carbohydrate: 37g

Dietary Fiber: 4g

Total Sugars: 32g

Protein: 1g

Total Fat: 1g

Saturated Fat: 0g

Vitamin A: 74IU

Vitamin C: 1mg

Folate: 9mcg

Sodium: 13mg

Calcium: 38mg

Iron: 1mg

Magnesium: 33mg

Potassium: 354mg

Ingredients

2 pitted Medjool dates

2 salted whole almonds

¼ teaspoon orange zest

Instructions

Stuff each date with an almond and roll in orange zest.

5.2 Instant-Pot Cashew Yogurt

Using an Instant Pot to make vegan yogurt at home is simple. You can prepare a batch of this creamy cashew yogurt in advance and have it ready for a quick breakfast or snack.

Preparation Information

Active Time:10 mins

Total Time:20 hrs 40 mins

Servings:8

Nutritional Information

Servings Per Recipe: 8

Serving Size: 1/2 cup

Calories: 233

Total Carbohydrate: 12g

Dietary Fiber: 4g

Total Sugars: 3g

Protein: 6g

Total Fat: 18g

Saturated Fat: 3g

Sodium: 4mg

Calcium: 37mg

Iron: 2mg

Magnesium: 1mg

Potassium: 1mg

Ingredients

2 ½ cups raw whole cashews

2 cups hot water (160℉ to 180℉)

4 cups tap water, divided

2 tablespoons tapioca flour

2 tablespoons vegan coconut-milk yogurt

Instructions

- Place cashews in a large heatproof bowl; cover with 2 cups hot water. Soak for 2 hours. Drain the cashews.

- Place the drained cashews in a blender; add 2 cups tap water. Process until smooth and creamy, 1 to 3 minutes, stopping to scrape down the sides as needed. Add tapioca flour and the remaining 2 cups tap water; process until very smooth and well combined, 1 to 3 minutes.

- Add the cashew milk to a programmable pressure multicooker (such as Instant Pot; times, instructions and settings may vary according to cooker brand or model). Lock the lid in place, turning the steam release handle to Venting position.

- Select Yogurt setting, and adjust to Boil or High (display may vary according to cooker brand or model). Select Start, if needed, to begin cooking (some models may start automatically). Cook until the milk reaches 180°F and the cooker beeps and reads Yogurt or End, about 30 minutes (for a thicker yogurt, see Tip).

- Remove the lid and the cooker insert. Let the milk cool to a temperature of 110°F to 116°F, about 1 hour. To speed up cooling, place the insert in a large bowl of ice water; let cool, stirring often. Do not allow the milk to cool below 110°F. (A skin may form on top; skim off with a small fine-mesh strainer or spoon, if needed, and discard.)

- Stir coconut-milk yogurt into the cooled milk. Return the insert to the cooker; lock the lid in place, turning the steam release handle to Venting position. Select Yogurt setting. Select Medium temperature for 10 hours.

- After 10 hours, open the lid carefully, minimizing condensation dripping onto the yogurt. Let the yogurt stand, undisturbed, until cooled to room temperature, about 1 hour. Cover with plastic wrap and refrigerate until completely chilled, at least 6 hours or up to 12 hours. (The consistency should be similar to a well-stirred, creamy salad dressing.)

- For thicker yogurt, line a fine-mesh strainer with a large coffee filter (or 2 pieces of cheesecloth) and set over a large bowl. Spoon in the yogurt. Refrigerate, covered with plastic wrap or a towel, until whey is strained from the yogurt and the yogurt is thick and creamy, at least 4 hours and up to 8 hours.

Tips

If your cooker has adjustable settings when using the Yogurt function, set to High or Boil, and set a timer for 5 minutes for a thicker, creamier yogurt. If a thinner consistency is desired, skip this step.

5.3 Crunchy Roasted Chickpeas

Try this satisfying snack instead of nuts. The tasty legumes are lower in calories and packed with fiber.

Preparation Information

Active Time:5 mins

Additional Time:30 mins

Total Time:35 mins

Servings:4

Yield:4 servings

Nutritional Information

Servings Per Recipe: 4

Serving Size: 1/4 cup

Calories: 100

Total Carbohydrate: 17g

Dietary Fiber: 5g

Total Sugars: 3g

Protein: 6g

Total Fat: 2g

Sodium: 170mg

Ingredients

1 (15 ounce) can no-salt-added chickpeas, rinsed

Nonstick cooking spray

¼ teaspoon sea salt

Instructions

Preheat the oven to 425°F. Pat chickpeas dry with paper towels; place on a large rimmed baking sheet. Coat with cooking spray and sprinkle with salt. Bake until crunchy, 30 to 45 minutes.

5.4 Sriracha-Buffalo Cauliflower Bites

This recipe for spicy Buffalo cauliflower bites is a great vegetarian alternative to Buffalo wings. Roasted cauliflower stands in for chicken and provides more fiber and fewer calories.

Preparation Information

Active Time:10 mins

Additional Time:20 mins

Total Time:25 mins

Servings:6

Yield:6 servings

Nutritional Information

Servings Per Recipe: 6

Serving Size: 3/4 cup

Calories: 99

Total Carbohydrate: 8g

Dietary Fiber: 3g

Total Sugars: 3g

Protein: 3g

Total Fat: 7g

Saturated Fat: 2g

Cholesterol: 5mg

Vitamin A: 169IU

Vitamin C: 70mg

Sodium: 288mg

Calcium: 33mg

Iron: 1mg

Potassium: 439mg

Ingredients

8 cups 1 1/2-inch cauliflower florets

2 tablespoons extra-virgin olive oil

¼ teaspoon kosher salt

2 tablespoons hot sauce, such as Frank's RedHot

1-2 tablespoons Sriracha

1 tablespoon butter, melted

1 tablespoon lemon juice

Instructions

- Preheat the oven to 450°F. Coat a large rimmed baking sheet with cooking spray.

- Toss cauliflower, oil and salt in a large bowl. Spread on the prepared baking sheet; reserve the bowl. Roast the cauliflower until it's starting to soften and brown on the bottom, about 15 minutes.

- Meanwhile, combine hot sauce, Sriracha to taste, butter and lemon juice in the large bowl. Add the roasted cauliflower and toss to coat. Return the cauliflower to the baking sheet and continue roasting until hot, about 5 minutes more.

5.5 Air-Fryer Crispy Chickpeas

Air-fried chickpea snacks are intensely flavored and incredibly crunchy. Drying the chickpeas is essential to a good crunch, so don't skip this step. If you have time, leave them out on the counter to dry for an hour or two before frying.

Preparation Information

Prep Time:20 mins

Total Time:20 mins

Servings:4

Yield:1 cup

Nutritional Information

Servings Per Recipe: 4

Serving Size: 1/4 cup

Calories: 132

Total Carbohydrate: 14g

Dietary Fiber: 3g

Protein: 5g

Total Fat: 6g

Saturated Fat: 1g

Vitamin A: 118IU

Vitamin C: 0mg

Folate: 0mcg

Sodium: 86mg

Calcium: 40mg

Iron: 1mg

Magnesium: 27mg

Potassium: 152mg

Ingredients

1 (15 ounce) can unsalted chickpeas, rinsed and drained

1 ½ tablespoons toasted sesame oil

¼ teaspoon smoked paprika

¼ teaspoon crushed red pepper

⅛ teaspoon salt

Cooking spray

2 lime wedges

Instructions

- Spread chickpeas on several layers of paper towels. Top with more paper towels and pat until very dry, rolling the chickpeas under the paper towels to dry all sides.

- Combine the chickpeas and oil in a medium bowl. Sprinkle it with paprika, crushed red pepper and salt. Pour into an air fryer basket and coat with cooking spray. Cook at 400 degrees F until very well browned, 12 to 14 minutes, shaking the basket occasionally. Squeeze lime wedges over the chickpeas and serve.

Chapter 6: Healthy Drinks

6.1 Green Juice

This nutritious green juice recipe is made with pears, celery, spinach, and parsley and is high in vitamin K, which supports healthy bones.

Preparation Information

Cook Time:15 mins

Total Time:15 mins

Servings:2

Yield:2 servings, about 8 ounces each

Nutritional Information

Servings Per Recipe: 2

Serving Size: about 8 ounces

Calories: 91

Total Carbohydrate: 20g

Dietary Fiber: 1g

Total Sugars: 15g

Protein: 1g

Total Fat: 1g

Saturated Fat: 0g

Vitamin A: 6132IU

Vitamin C: 51mg

Folate: 174mcg

Sodium: 192mg

Calcium: 136mg

Iron: 3mg

Magnesium: 71mg

Potassium: 409mg

Ingredients

½ cup fresh parsley

3 cups spinach

½ lemon, peeled

2 medium pears, cut into eighths

6 large stalks celery, trimmed

Ice cubes (optional)

Instructions

- Working in this order, process parsley, spinach, lemon, pears and celery through a juicer according to the manufacturer's directions. (No juicer? See Tip.)

- Fill 2 glasses with ice, if desired, and pour the juice into the glasses. Serve immediately.

Tips

No juicer? No problem. Try this DIY version of blended and strained juice instead: Coarsely chop all ingredients. First, place the soft and/or juice ingredients in the blender and process until liquefied. Then, add the remaining ingredients; blend until liquefied. Cut two 24-inch-long pieces of cheesecloth. Completely unfold each piece and then stack the pieces on top of each other. Fold the double stack in half so you have a 4-layer stack of cloth. Line a large bowl with the cheesecloth and pour the contents of the blender into the center. Gather the edges of the cloth together in one hand and use the other hand to twist and squeeze the bundle to extract all the juice from the pulp. Wear a pair of rubber gloves if you don't want the juice to stain your hands.

6.2 Anti-Inflammatory Golden Tonic

The momentum behind functional foods and wellness elixirs is at an all-time high. Expensive products are touted as having the power to do everything from restoring gut health to boosting immunity and fighting inflammation, but their health claims are often backed by little solid science. So instead of pricey supplements, we're mixing up a more affordable antidote that's both healthy and homemade. A tonic, by definition, is a combination of ingredients that have the potential to enhance or restore health. While this tonic (or any tonic) is not a cure-all remedy, consuming more anti-inflammatory foods—like the ones found in this tonic—over time may only not only ease current symptoms (such as fatigue, joint pain and chronic bloating), but it may also reduce the risk of future diseases and slow aging. The combination of green tea, herbs, honey, apple-cider vinegar and spices also makes for a tasty and refreshing beverage

Preparation Information

Prep Time:10 mins

Additional Time:1 hr 15 mins

Total Time:1 hr 25 mins

Servings:4

Yield:4 cups

Nutritional Information

Servings Per Recipe: 4

Serving Size: 1 cup

Calories: 18

Total Carbohydrate: 5g
Dietary Fiber: 0g
Total Sugars: 4g
Added Sugars: 4g
Protein: 0g
Vitamin A: 19IU
Folate: 0 mcg
Sodium: 4mg
Calcium: 6mg
Iron: 0mg
Magnesium: 3mg
Potassium: 23 mg

Ingredients

2 cups filtered water
2 bags green tea
5 sprigs fresh thyme, lightly bruised with the side of a knife

1 (2 inch) piece peeled ginger, finely grated
1 (2 inch) piece peeled turmeric, finely grated
1 tablespoon honey, preferably manuka
1 tablespoon raw unfiltered cider vinegar
Ice cubes
2 cups chilled sparkling water
Lime wedges for serving

Instructions

- Bring filtered water to a gentle simmer in a small saucepan over medium-high heat. Add tea bags, thyme, ginger, turmeric, honey and vinegar, stirring to dissolve the honey. Reduce heat to low and let the mixture steep for 15 minutes. Strain through a fine-mesh sieve into a mason jar. Refrigerate for 1 hour.

- Fill 4 glasses half full of ice. Divide the tonic mixture evenly among the glasses (about 1/2 cup tonic per glass). Top each with 1/2 cup sparkling water. Serve with a lime wedge, if desired.

6.3 Ginger-Turmeric-Carrot Shots

The crispness of the fresh ginger and the sweetness of the carrots and coconut water are captured in this cool picture. This would be simple to double and store in your refrigerator, ready for whenever you are, if your blender is large enough.

Nutritional Information

Servings Per Recipe: 4

Serving Size: 2 oz.

Calories: 59

Total Carbohydrate: 14g

Dietary Fiber: 3g

Total Sugars: 7g

Protein: 1g

Total Fat: 0g

Saturated Fat: 0g

Vitamin A: 18944IU

Vitamin C: 11mg

Folate: 22mcg

Sodium: 127mg

Calcium: 42mg

Iron: 1mg

Magnesium: 18mg

Potassium: 471mg

Ingredients

1 pound carrots, very coarsely chopped

1 (2 inch) piece fresh turmeric, peeled and coarsely chopped

1 (2 inch) piece fresh ginger, peeled and coarsely chopped

¾ cup unsweetened coconut water, divided

Pinch of salt

Instructions

- Process carrots, turmeric, ginger and 1/2 cup coconut water in a blender on high speed until completely smooth, about 2 minutes. Pour the mixture through a fine-mesh strainer into a clean jar or container, pressing lightly with a rubber spatula to extract juice; discard solids.

- Stir in salt and the remaining 1/4 cup coconut water.

6.4 Apple Cider Vinegar Tonic

While this weight-loss tonic won't instantly help you adopt healthy behaviors, it might help you lose weight. The sour taste (the acetic acid) in apple cider vinegar may help you eat less and feel fuller for longer. Caffeine and antioxidants included in green tea may assist fat loss. You may be able to burn more calories with ginger. Additionally, maple syrup gives this hydrating beverage a hint of natural sweetness. To help you lose weight, add this tonic to your diet along with prudent food and exercise.

Preparation Information

Prep Time:5 mins

Total Time:5 mins

Servings:1

Yield:1 cup

Nutritional Information

Servings Per Recipe: 1

Serving Size: 1 cup

Calories: 22

Total Carbohydrate: 5g

Total Sugars: 4g

Added Sugars: 4g

Vitamin C: 0mg

Folate: 0 mcg

Sodium: 2mg

Calcium: 8mg

Iron: 0mg

Magnesium: 3mg

Potassium: 58mg

Ingredients

1 cup brewed green tea, chilled

1 tablespoon raw cider vinegar

1 teaspoon pure maple syrup

1 teaspoon grated fresh ginger

Lemon wedge (optional)

Instructions

Stir tea, vinegar, syrup and ginger in a medium glass. Add a squeeze of lemon, if desired.

6.5 Elderberry Elixir Mocktail

This effervescent winter mocktail features immune-supporting elderberry syrup alongside anti-inflammatory turmeric and a dose of vitamin C from orange juice. Use freshly squeezed orange juice for the best flavor. Depending on the sweetness of your elderberry syrup, you may want to use more or a little less.

Preparation Information

Active Time:5 mins
Total Time:5 mins
Servings:1

Nutritional Information

Servings Per Recipe: 1
Serving Size: 1 mocktail
Calories: 124

Total Carbohydrate: 29g
Total Sugars: 24g
Protein: 1g
Vitamin A: 125IU

Sodium: 1mg

Ingredients

2 ounces freshly squeezed orange juice

1 ounce elderberry syrup (see Tip)

½ ounce freshly squeezed lemon juice

¼ teaspoon ground turmeric, or more to taste

Ice

Sparkling water

Orange slice for garnish

Instructions

- Combine orange juice, elderberry syrup, lemon juice and turmeric in a cocktail shaker. Add ice to make the shaker 3/4 full. Cover and shake until chilled, then strain into a rocks glass filled with ice. (Alternatively, for a layered look, shake the citrus juices and turmeric and strain into a glass filled with crushed ice. Drizzle the elderberry syrup over the ice.)

- Top with sparkling water and garnish with an orange slice, if desired.

Chapter 7: Vegetarian Recipes

7.1 Vegan Lentil Soup

This vegan lentil soup recipe is packed with fresh ingredients and plenty of lentils that deliver a healthy dose of fiber in each bite. This vegan soup is the perfect cold-weather lunch or healthy dinner the whole family will love.

Preparation Information

Active Time:20 mins

Total Time:1 hr

Servings:6

Nutritional Information

Servings Per Recipe: 6

Serving Size: about 1 cup

Calories: 272

Total Carbohydrate: 42g

Dietary Fiber: 9g

Protein: 13g

Total Fat: 7g

Saturated Fat: 1g

Vitamin A: 4618IU

Sodium: 487 mg

Ingredients

2 tablespoons extra-virgin olive oil

1 ½ cups chopped yellow onions

1 cup chopped carrots

3 cloves garlic, minced

2 tablespoons no-salt-added tomato paste

4 cups reduced-sodium vegetable broth

1 cup water

1 (15 ounce) can no-salt-added cannellini beans, rinsed

1 cup mixed dry lentils (brown, green and black)

½ cup chopped sun-dried tomatoes in oil, drained

¾ teaspoon salt

½ teaspoon ground pepper

1 tablespoon chopped fresh dill, plus more for garnish

1 ½ teaspoons red-wine vinegar

Instructions

- Heat oil in a large, heavy pot over medium heat. Add onions and carrots; cook, stirring occasionally, until softened, 3 to 4 minutes. Add garlic and cook, stirring constantly, until fragrant, about 1 minute. Add tomato paste and cook, stirring constantly, until the mixture is evenly coated, about 1 minute.

- Stir in broth, water, cannellini beans, lentils, sun-dried tomatoes, salt and pepper. Bring to a boil over medium-high heat; reduce heat to medium-low to maintain a simmer. Cover and simmer until the lentils are tender, 30 to 40 minutes.

- Remove from heat and stir in dill and vinegar. Garnish with additional dill, if desired, and serve.

7.2 Frittata with Asparagus, Leek & Ricotta

Serve this spring-vegetable-loaded frittata with an arugula salad and a hunk of crusty bread. Tip: This recipe cooks quickly, so be sure to have all your ingredients prepped and ready to go.

Preparation Information

Active Time:20 mins

Total Time:20 mins

Servings:4

Nutritional Information

Servings Per Recipe: 4

Serving Size: 1 slice

Calories: 369

Total Carbohydrate: 14g

Dietary Fiber: 3g

Total Sugars: 5g

Protein: 18g

Total Fat: 27g

Saturated Fat: 9g

Cholesterol: 389mg

Vitamin A: 2445IU

Vitamin C: 12mg

Vitamin D: 83IU

Vitamin E: 4mg

Folate: 127mcg

Vitamin K: 83mcg

Sodium: 549mg

Iron: 5mg

Magnesium: 47mg

Potassium: 424mg

Zinc: 2mg

Vitamin B12: 1mcg

Ingredients

8 large eggs

¼ cup crème fraîche

½ teaspoon salt

¼ teaspoon ground pepper

2 tablespoons extra-virgin olive oil

3 cups thinly sliced leeks (about 2 medium), rinsed well and patted dry

1 pound asparagus, trimmed and cut into 1-inch pieces

¼ cup part-skim ricotta

2 tablespoons pesto

¼ cup fresh basil

Instructions

- Position rack in upper third of oven; preheat broiler.

- Whisk eggs, crème fraîche, salt and pepper in a medium bowl; set near the stove. Heat oil in a large cast-iron skillet over medium-high heat. Add leeks and asparagus and cook, stirring frequently, until soft, 5 to 6 minutes.

- Pour the egg mixture over the vegetables and cook, lifting the edges so the uncooked egg can flow underneath, until nearly set, about 2 minutes. Dollop ricotta and pesto on top and place the pan under the broiler until the eggs are slightly browned, 1 1/2 to 2 minutes. Let stand for 3 minutes.

- Run a spatula around the edge of the frittata, then underneath, until you can slide or lift it out onto a cutting board or serving plate. Top with basil.

7.3 Guacamole Chopped Salad

All of the delicious guacamole flavors you love in a healthy veggie-packed salad. Want to pump up the protein? Add leftover roast chicken or sautéed shrimp. Serve with tortilla chips on the side (or crumbled over the top) to take it up a notch.

Preparation Information

Prep Time:20 mins

Total Time:20 mins

Servings:4

Yield:4 servings

Nutritional Information

Servings Per Recipe: 4

Serving Size: 1 1/3 cups

Calories: 245

Total Carbohydrate: 13g

Dietary Fiber: 8g

Total Sugars: 3g

Protein: 3g

Total Fat: 22g

Saturated Fat: 3g

Vitamin A: 4570IU

Vitamin C 20mg

Folate: 153 mcg

Sodium: 185mg

Calcium: 36mg

Iron: 1mg

Magnesium: 42mg

Potassium: 720mg

Ingredients

2 tablespoons corn oil or avocado oil

2 tablespoons lime juice

1 clove garlic, grated

¼ teaspoon salt

¼ teaspoon ground pepper

4 cups chopped romaine lettuce

2 ripe avocados, diced

1 cup grape tomatoes, quartered

¼ cup slivered red onion

1 tablespoon chopped pickled jalapeño pepper

Instructions

- Whisk oil, lime juice, garlic, salt and pepper in a large bowl. Add romaine, avocado, tomatoes, onion and jalapeño; toss gently to coat.

7.4 Chhole (Chickpea Curry)

This healthy Indian recipe is a flavorful chickpea curry that you can make in just 20 minutes. Also called chana masala, this dish is a comforting and delicious dinner.

Preparation Information

Active Time:15 mins

Total Time:20 mins

Servings:6

Yield:6 servings

Nutritional Information

Servings Per Recipe: 6

Serving Size about: 1 cup

Calories: 278

Total Carbohydrate: 30g

Dietary Fiber: 6g

Total Sugars: 3g

Protein: 6g

Total Fat: 16g

Saturated Fat: 1g

Vitamin A: 260 IU

Vitamin C: 18mg

Folate: 75mcg

Sodium: 354mg

Calcium: 65mg

Iron: 2mg

Magnesium: 34mg

Potassium: 356mg

Ingredients

1 medium serrano pepper, cut into thirds

4 large cloves garlic

1 2-inch piece fresh ginger, peeled and coarsely chopped

1 medium yellow onion, chopped (1-inch)

6 tablespoons canola oil or grapeseed oil

2 teaspoons ground coriander

2 teaspoons ground cumin

½ teaspoon ground turmeric

2 ¼ cups no-salt-added canned diced tomatoes with their juice (from a 28-ounce can)

¾ teaspoon kosher salt

2 15-ounce cans chickpeas, rinsed

2 teaspoons garam masala

Fresh cilantro for garnish

Instructions

- Pulse serrano, garlic and ginger in a food processor until minced. Scrape down the sides and pulse again. Add onion; pulse until finely chopped, but not watery.

- Heat oil in a large saucepan over medium-high heat. Add the onion mixture and cook, stirring occasionally, until softened, 3 to 5 minutes. Add coriander, cumin and turmeric and cook, stirring, for 2 minutes.

- Pulse tomatoes in the food processor until finely chopped. Add to the pan along with salt. Reduce heat to maintain a simmer and cook, stirring occasionally, for 4 minutes. Add chickpeas and garam masala, reduce heat to a gentle simmer, cover and cook, stirring occasionally, for 5 minutes more. Serve topped with cilantro, if desired.

7.5 Quinoa-Black Bean Salad

Enjoy this quinoa and black bean salad as a delicious and quick vegetarian main dish or as a side for grilled chicken or steak. And don't forget the leftovers! They make an easy lunch on the go.

Preparation Information

Prep Time:20 mins

Total Time:20 mins

Servings:6

Yield:9 cups

Nutritional Information

Servings Per Recipe: 6

Serving Size: 1 1/2 cups

Calories: 458

Total Carbohydrate: 47g

Dietary Fiber: 10g

Total Sugars: 7g

Protein: 14g

Total Fat: 26g

Saturated Fat: 6g

Cholesterol: 15mg

Vitamin A: 785IU

Vitamin C: 18mg

Folate: 101mcg

Sodium: 440mg

Calcium: 204mg

Iron: 4mg

Magnesium: 136mg

Potassium: 746mg

Ingredients

2 ears corn, husks removed

1 medium zucchini, cut lengthwise into 1/4-inch planks

6 tablespoons extra-virgin olive oil

¼ cup lime juice

1 ½ teaspoons ground cumin

3 cups cooked quinoa (see Associated Recipes)

3 cups baby arugula

1 (15 ounce) can no-salt-added black beans, rinsed

1 cup pico de gallo, divided

½ cup chopped fresh cilantro, divided

¾ cup crumbled cotija cheese, divided

1 avocado, diced, divided

Instructions

Preheat a gas grill or charcoal grill to medium (350-400 degrees F). Grill corn, uncovered and turning occasionally, until tender and charred on all sides, about 10 minutes. Grill zucchini, uncovered and turning once, until charred and tender, about 2 minutes per side. (Alternatively, heat a grill pan coated with cooking spray over medium-high heat. Grill corn, turning occasionally, until charred and tender, 4 to 5 minutes. Grill zucchini, turning once, until charred and tender, about 2 minutes per side.) Coarsely chop zucchini and cut kernels from the cobs.

Whisk oil, lime juice and cumin in a large bowl. Add the zucchini, the corn, quinoa, arugula, beans and half each of pico de gallo, cilantro, cheese and avocado. Gently toss to combine.

Top with the remaining pico de gallo, cilantro, cheese and avocado.

To make ahead

Prepare salad as directed, omitting avocado. Cover and refrigerate for up to 3 days. Add avocado just before serving.

Review

Dear readers, thank you for your support and interest in "The Easy Anti-inflammatory Diet". We hope you enjoyed exploring our collection of recipes! Your feedback is incredibly valuable to us as we strive to continuously improve and provide you with the best possible experience. If you've tried any of our recipes, we'd love to hear about your thoughts and experiences. Please take a moment to share your review and let us know how we're doing. Your input helps us tailor our offerings to better meet your needs and preferences. Thank you for being a part of our community, and we look forward to hearing from you!

9 798325 851995